Essential Oils:

Beginner's Guide To Losing Weight Fast Using Essential Oils

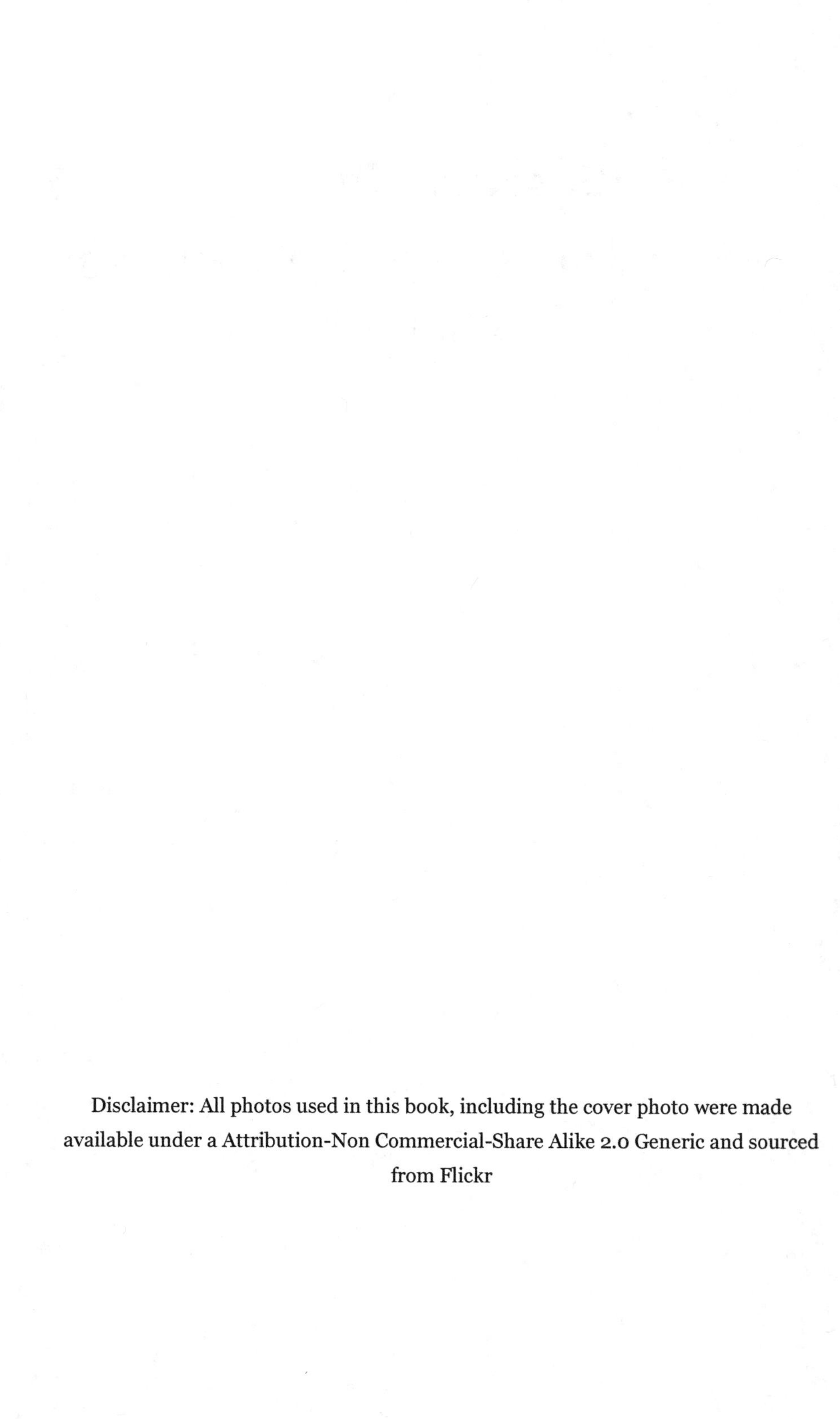

Table of content:

Introduction - You've tried everything...

You've followed the advice of doctors, nutritionists, and started eating right and exercising, but you feel you can boost what you're doing with essential oils. So, you go online and look for information, finding everything from how essential oils don't work to websites that list oils that DO work, but not how to use them. You want to use natural ways of smoothing and toning as well as burning fat, but all the information has you scratching your head. You're in luck! This book has been made easy to follow, understand, and yes, we even have recipes you can try out! So, if you're ready, what are you waiting for?

Chapter 1 - The Basics

You've seen the bottles online and in health stores, but you're wondering how they are made and how they work. Essential oils are the purest, and most potent, form of the herb, flower, or plant in general, but not all plants can produce essential oils. There are more than 90 different essential oils on the market, and not all of them are recommended for layman's use.

Through distillation, the oil is expressed and cooled then placed into dark glass bottles for distribution. The form of natural medicine you need essential oils for is called Aromatherapy. Think for a moment. When you were little and you walked into your home and smelled cookies, you smiled. They made you happy and you couldn't wait until you could eat some. When you caught a whiff of peppermint, you instantly felt relaxed yet ready to focus on your task. That's aromatherapy, and it has a myriad of uses.

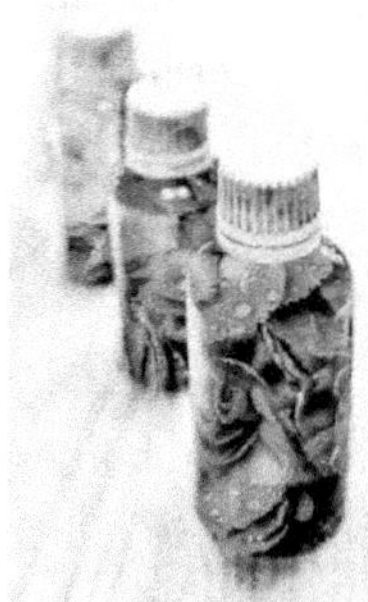

There are a few things to keep in mind when handling essential oils.

1. Do not use them undiluted. There are websites out there which try to convince you that therapeutic grade essential oils are fine to ingest and use undiluted. This is wrong. Even Lavender, which is the only exception to this rule can give you contact dermatitis when used too often undiluted. Essential oils are toxic when ingested without diluting them in food.

2. Use gloves when handling essential oils. This is because they all can cause contact dermatitis.

3. Be sure you are not allergic to the oils you intend to use. This should be basic information and not really needed to put in a book, but it is important to note. If you are allergic to a plant, you can also be allergic to a related medicinal plant through it's classification.

4. Keep all essential oils in a dark cool place. Extreme heat can make them evaporate in the bottles they are stored in.

5. Keep them out of the reach of children. Essentials oils are a great way to be healthy, but they are toxic when ingested.

6. Make sure you are not allergic to the oils. Doing a patch test can help with this. Take three drops of essential oil in 1 teaspoon of base oil and rub it into a small patch of skin. If within 24 you have not had a reaction, you are not allergic. It is better, however, if you go to an allergist to have the test done.

Blending and Preparations

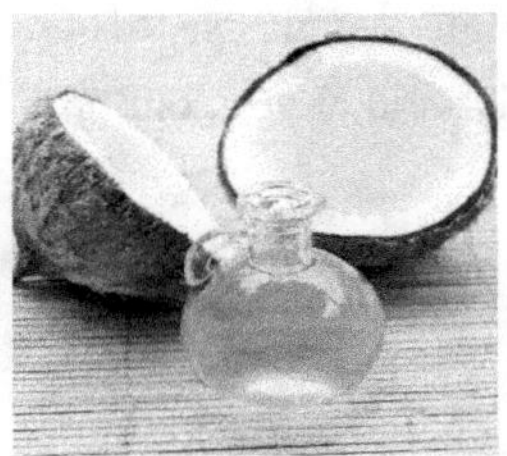

When you blend essential oils for preparations, there are base oils you add them to in a lot of cases. Here is a list of the most popular ones.

Almond Oil, Sweet

This is the most popular oil to use in blends for Aromatherapy. It is a light, relatively odorless oil, that is packed with vitamin E, Vitamin K, and the omega fatty acid 6 and 9. It is recommended for all skin types, but if you are allergic to tree nuts, there are alternatives.

Apricot Kernel Oil

This is the go-to alternate oil for those with tree nut allergies. It is packed with Vitamin E and the same fatty acids as Sweet Almond Oil above. This oils is also good for all skin types, even sensitive skin. You may still need to do a skin test to make sure you are not allergic.

Argan Oil

You've seen this oil in smoothing tonics for hair and shampoos to prevent frizzing. It's good for all skin types, even aging and prematurely aging skin. It's packed with the same vitamins and fatty acids as Apricot above. It can be used by itself, but when used in blends with other base oils, 15%-20% max is best.

Coconut Oil

This oil can be used 100% in solo blends and 30%-50% in blends with other carrier oils. It contains Lauric acid, which is a saturated fatty acid). Many people use this for mature skin and dry skin. The most popular form of this oil is solid at 76F, but does melt under low heat without losing any of its properties.

Grapeseed Oil

The cold-pressed oil is the form that is used in Aromatherapy as it is the most pure form of the oil and it can be used without having to mix it with other base oils. It's safe for all skin types and especially good for oily skin and skin prone to acne breakouts.

Jojoba Oil

This is technically a wax, but it can be used without being diluted. It's recommended for all skin types including sensitive skin. When combining it with other base oils a 30%-80% concentration is often used. It contains 3, 6, and 9 Omega Fatty acids as well as Vitamin E.

Safflower Oil

This has become popular in cooking, but it can also be used in Aromatherapy blends by itself and in 30%-50% concentrations when you blend it with other base oils. It is good for all skin types and comes recommended for mature skin and acne-prone skin, too.

Sunflower oil

This has softening and moisturizing properties. It can be used without diluting or in concentrations of 30%-70%. It is good for all skin types. And contains the same nutrients as Apricot Seed oil.

Now we get to the stronger carrier oils, the ones you need to dilute. I am not listing all the oils used, just the more affordable ones.

Avocado Oil

This is generally used in concentrations of 10%-40%. It contains vitamins A, B, D, and E as well as the Omega fatty acids 3, 6, 9. This makes it great for all skins types. You can use it undiluted, but it has a strong aroma and that is one of the reasons why it is part of a mixture.

Evening Primrose Oil

This is an oil that is used in concentrations of 10%-30%. It nourishes all skin types and has a high amount of Omega 3, 6, and 9 fatty acids as well as gamma linolenic acid.

Olive Oil

This is on oil that is used in cooking but also in concentrations of 30%-50% in base oil blends. It's good for all skin types but especially good with mature skin types.

This list will be shorter than the actual list of all the ways you can prepare essential oils to make it more tailored to helping you lose weight.

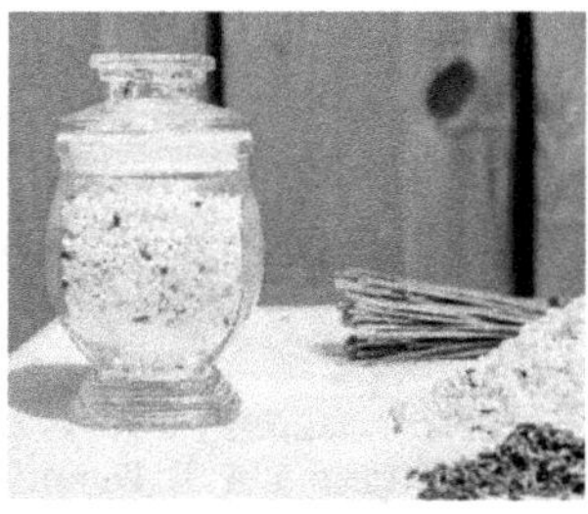

Bath Salts/Mineral Baths

These can help relax you and balance your hormones, moods and also help to stimulate your metabolism depending on what essential oils you use. There are two base recipes for mineral oils.

Base Recipe I

1 1/2 Cup Epsom Salts
1/4 Cup Baking Soda
1/4 Cup Borax
1/2 Cup Sea Salt

Base Recipe II

1 1/2 Cup Magnesium Salts
1/2 Cup Sea Salt
1/2 Cup Borax

Diffuser Blend

This is a blend of undiluted essential oils that can be used in a diffuser.

Inhalers

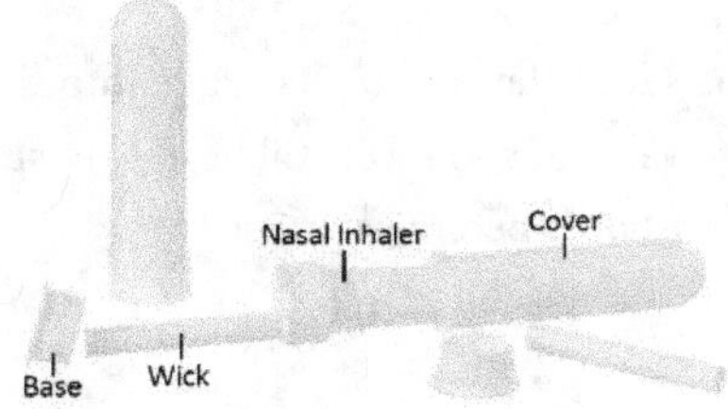

This is a way of delivering a quick inhale of essential oils without having to carry around a diffuser. You use undiluted essential oil blends.

Making Inhalers

Place 15 drops of an essential oil blend onto a small plate. Using tweezers, roll the wick around in the blend until all the blend is absorbed, and assemble the inhaler.

Lotions

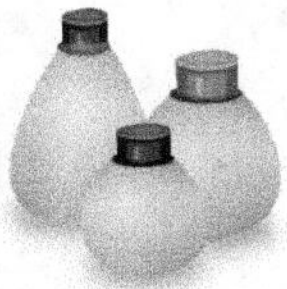

You can buy lotion base to make this types of preparation. You blend the essential oils into the lotion base.

Ointments

Ointments are think and help to keep the essential oils in contact with the skin longer.

2 cups Almond or Olive Oil
1/4 cup beeswax

In a double boiler add the oil and the beeswax until the wax melts. Pour into the container of your choice and allow it to become warm but you will still be able to stir it. Add the essential oils and mix well. Let it sit 24-hours before use.

Massage oils/Roll-Ons

This is a mixture of base/carrier oils and essential oils. It is used by massaging the oil into the muscles or close to the glands topically. The small roll-on bottle makes the massage oil convenient in that you can roll the oil onto the area, give it a few circular massages, and you're ready to take on the day.

Sugar Scrubs

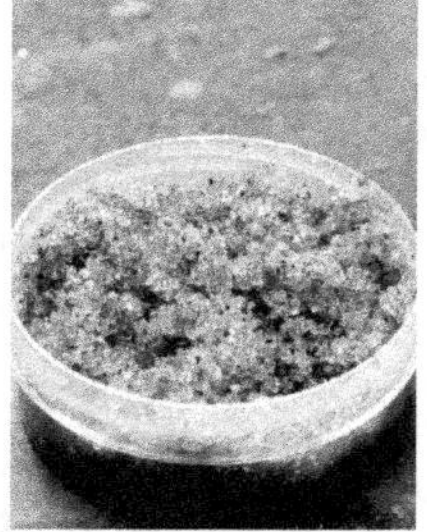

These are a good way to cleanse and exfoliate the skin. It also a good way to apply essential oils to a more remote location.

Base Recipe

1/2 Cup Brown Sugar

1/2 Cup Olive oil or coconut oil

Tools of the Trade

In every hobby, trade, or craft, there are tools you will need and Aromatherapy is no different. Here is a list of things you will need to mix, measure, and store your blends. Surprisingly enough, many of the things on this list you already have in your kitchen.

Mixing Bowls

Glass mixing bowls are best so as not to leech the properties of metal bowls into your blends. Generally, you will need small to medium sized bowls.

Food Scale

You can more accurately measure ingredients needed for your preparations with this.

Measuring spoons and cups

Measuring out liquids is key and using these will make it a lot easier. Again, try to avoid metal tools for this.

Funnel

Most of the preparations will be in liquid form. A funnel will help you pour the recipes into bottles for storage.

Double Boiler

There will be times you will need to melt ingredients without them coming in contact with water. If you can find a glass double boiler, that would be best. If not, you can use a glass mixing bowl and place it in the pot with the water.

Blender/Mixer

Sometimes you will need to mix the ingredients well, and this will come in handy.

Bottles and Lidded Containers

You will need dark glass or plastic bottles to reduce the amount of sunlight that hits the blends you make. Lidded containers are for sugar and salt scrubs.

Diffuser/Candle warmer/Potpourri warmer

You can use undiluted essential oils in diffusers designed to release the fragrance into the air; however, diffusers can be a little heavy on the budget.

You can, instead, invest in a candle warmer or potpourri warmer to put the essential blends into. All you need is ten drop of the undiluted blends on either, and it will proficiently fill a moderately sized master bedroom with fragrance.

Labels and a recipe book

You will need to label your finish products to keep things organized and keep track of when they expire, or lose a lot of their potency. As you experiment with your own recipes, you will need a book or small file box to keep them in for future use.

Baking Soda, Sea Salt, Epsom Salts, Borax

These are four ingredients you will need for making mineral bath salts.

Beeswax

This is an ingredient often used in ointments and balms to help them harden and add nutrients to the blend.

Chapter 2 - The Essential Oils

When you look at the essential oils from their medicinal properties, they can help with everything from elevating our mood, to helping your body heal, and beyond. Smelling certain essential blends will reduce your appetite. The following list of essential oils will have their Latin names included because one common name can refer to two or three different essential oils.

Bergamot (Citrus bergamia)

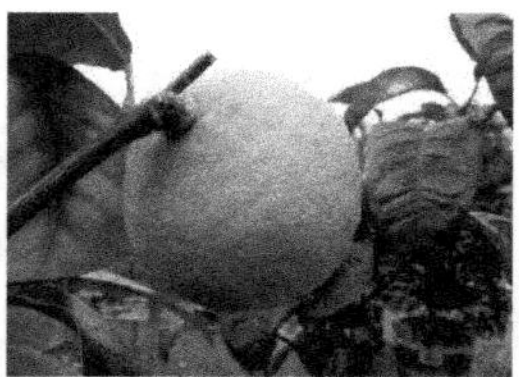

This citrus essential oil strengthen your emotions and helps with depression and stress. This is often good to use during weight loss because your emotional state needs to be in a good place to help you lose weight and keep it off. The only thing to be careful of is going out in the sun directly after a blend with bergamot in it. It can cause sensitivity to the sun.

Carrot Seed (Daucus carota)

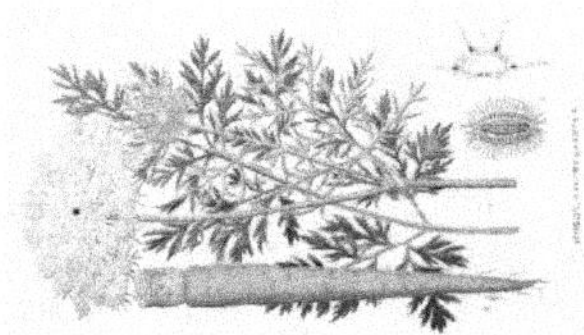

This essential oil is used in cases of sensitive skin and can help with water retention. Best avoided during pregnancy and breastfeeding.

Cedarwood, Virginia (Juniperus virginiana)

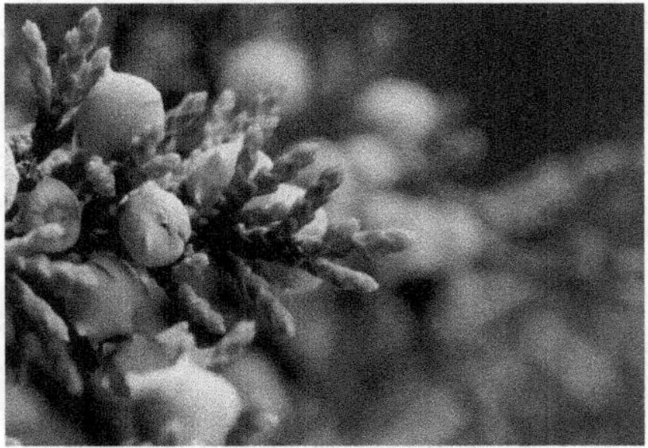

This oil is good for helping prevent water retention and is also good for smoothing cellulite. Can cause skin irritation.

Cinnamon (Cinnamomum zeylanicum)

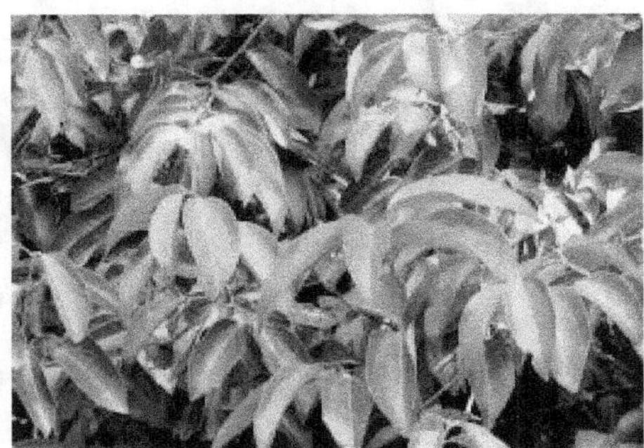

This is the leaf of the tree. The bark is too volatile to use. It helps maintain you energy levels, which comes in handy before or during workouts or for a long day at work. It helps to combat fatigue. Avoid if you are taking blood thinners, are pregnant or breast feeding or have overly sensitive skin.

Coriander Seed (Coriandrum sativum)

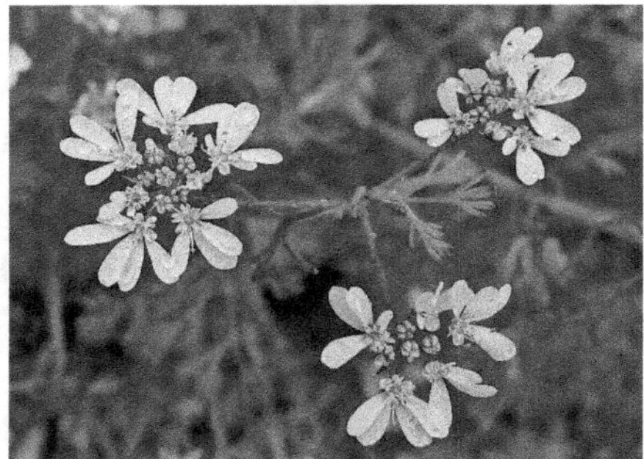

This essential oil is good for all types of digestive problems and disorders. It helps to detoxify cells and aids in fighting mental fatigue.

Cypress (Cupressus sempervirens)

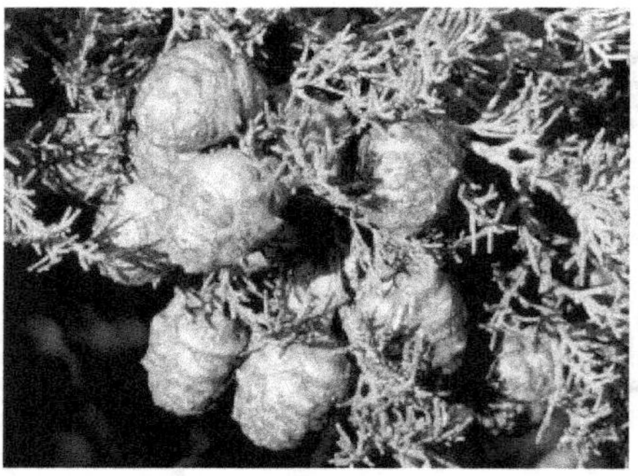

This helps with circulation issues which can hamper exercise and helping to prevent the retention of fluid. Avoid using this one too often, and avoid altogether if you are pregnant or breastfeeding.

Eucalyptus Peppermint (Eucalyptus dives)

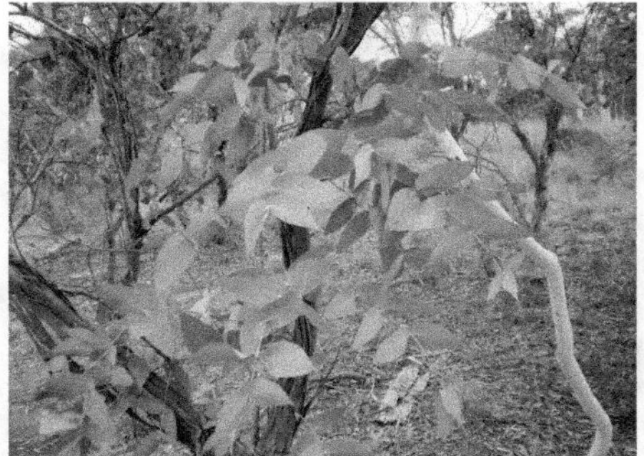

There are four different kinds of Eucalyptus. This one can help the body smooth out bumps due to cellulite. It also helps fight fatigue and exhaustion. Please, avoid this essential oil if you are pregnant.

Fennel (Foeniculum vulgare)

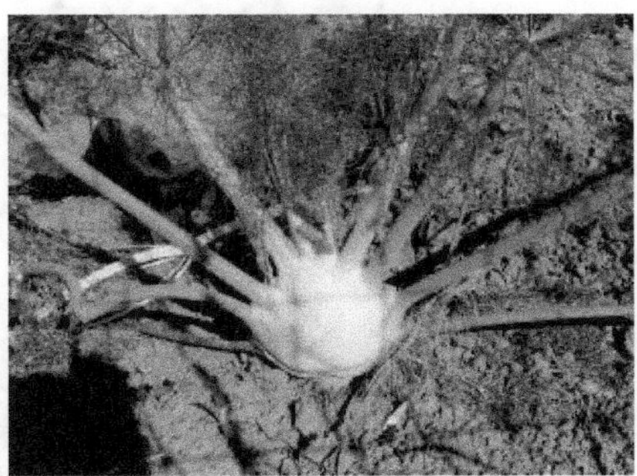

This essential oil comes in handy when you want to smooth cellulite or help your body correct water retention. It also helps with digestive issues which can prevent your body from absorbing nutrients.

Don't use if you are taking a lot of prescription medications. Avoid if pregnant or breastfeeding.

Frankincense (Boswellia carteri)

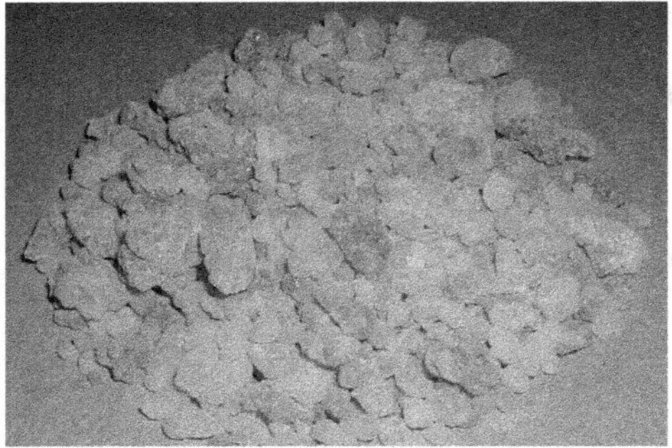

Since stubborn fat tends to hang around because of stress, this essential oil helps in that regard. It also helps with mental fatigue.

Ginger (Zingiber officinale)

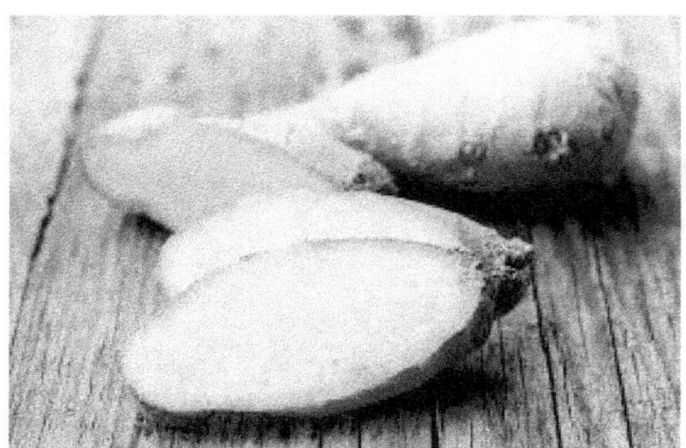

This is an immune booster that can also stimulate the body as a whole. Ginger is also good to add to blends as a catalyst.

Grapefruit (Citrus paradisi)

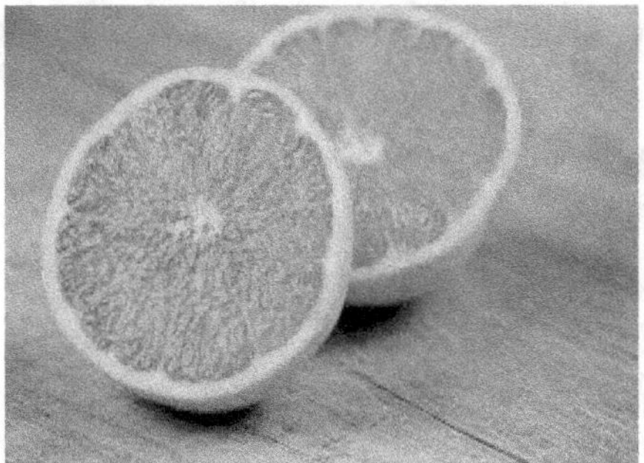

This essential oil is recommended when you're trying to lose weight, smooth out cellulite, purge any retained fluids, and it even helps to keep your spirits up. Try not to use it if you are taking multiple prescription medications.

Greenland Moss (Ledum groenlandicum)

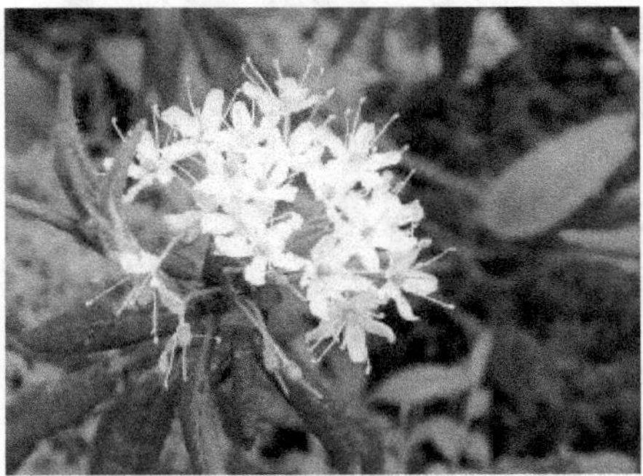

This little known essential oil helps to promote a healthy liver, helps to boost the body during weight loss, and helps to prevent water retention.

Jasmine (Jasminum grandiforum)

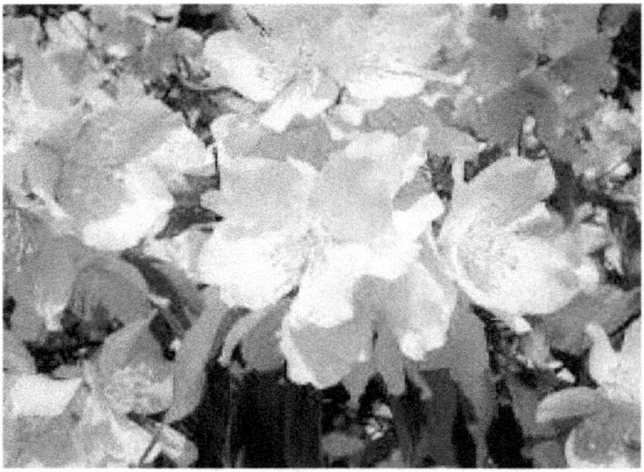

This oil is used in weight loss blends to help with stress, feelings of low self-esteem, and fatigue.

Lemon (Citrus limon)

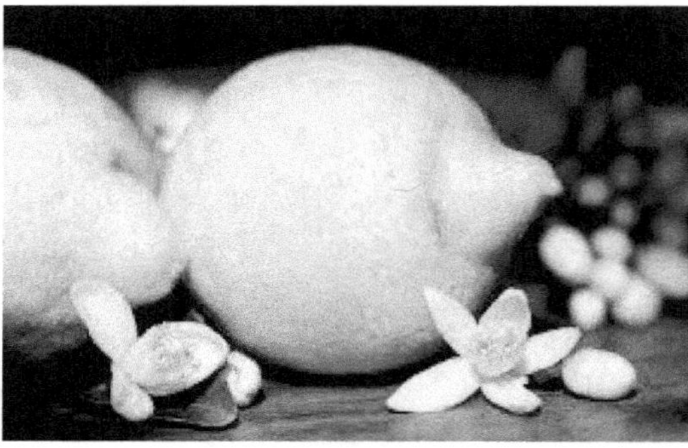

This oils helps with digestive problems. It helps to detox cells, and also helps the body to get rid of cellulite.

Lemongrass (Cymbopogon flexuosus)

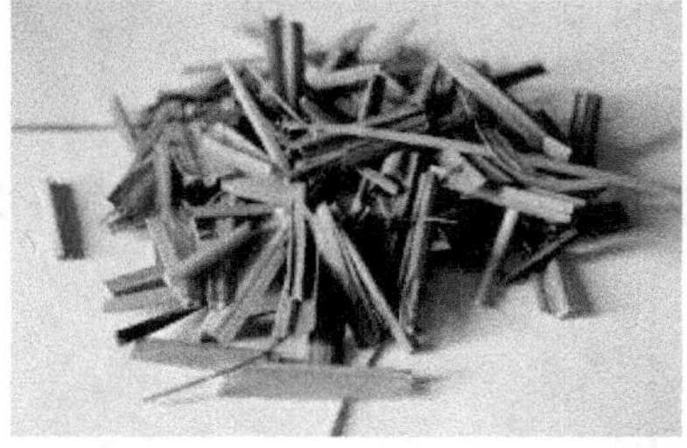

This detoxifying essential oil can also help smooth cellulite and as well helps with exhaustion.

Lime (Citrus auranifolia)

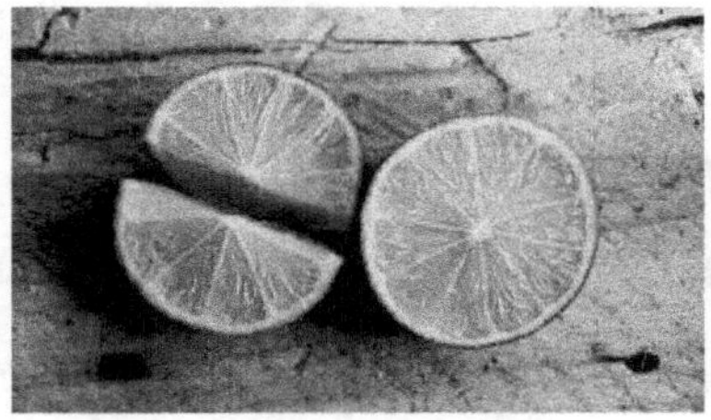

Helps with loss of appetite, detoxifies, and helps to smooth cellulite.

Mandarin (Citrus reticulata)

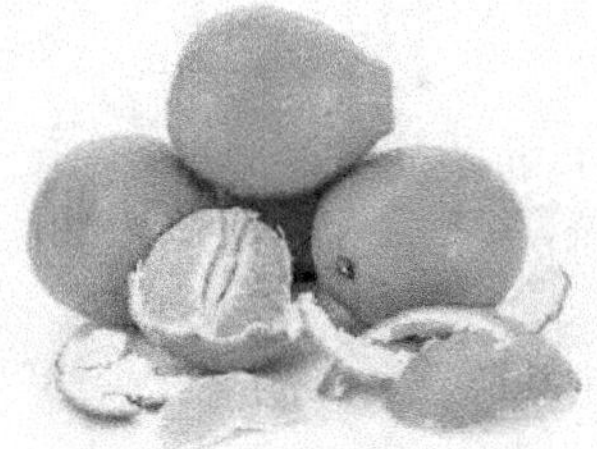

This helps with cellulite and digestive disorders.

Orange (Citrus sinesis)

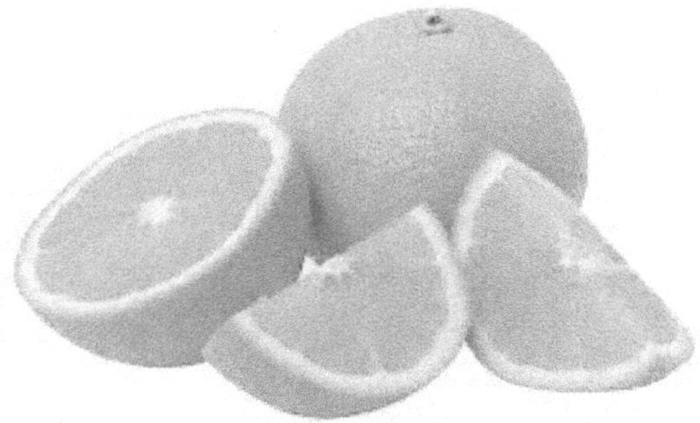

This helps with retention of fluid, smooths cellulite, and helps to raise spirits and stress.

Peppermint (Mentha piperita)

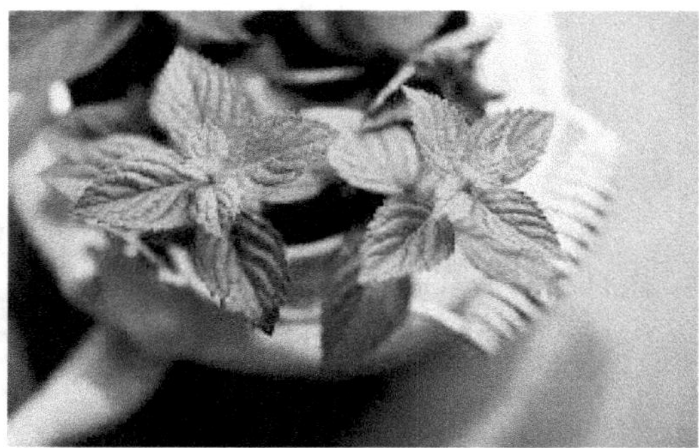

It helps with all sorts of digestive problems that can prevent proper weight loss. It can also help with fatigue. Avoid in early stages of pregnancy.

Rosemary (Rosmarius officinalis)

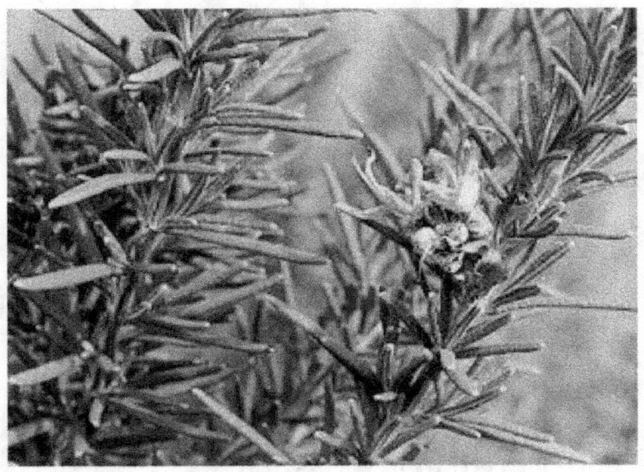

This essential oil is recommended for smoothing cellulite, improving circulation. It also helps to detoxify cells, too. Avoid if pregnant.

Saro (Cinnamosma fragrans)

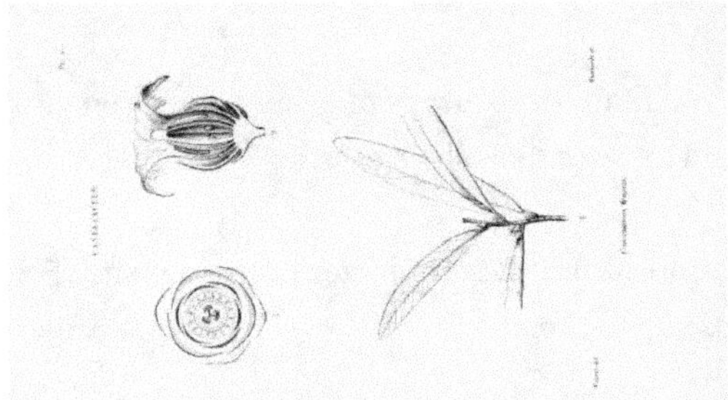

This is another little known essential oil on the mass market, but it comes in handy when smoothing cellulite.

Violet Leaf (Viola odorata)

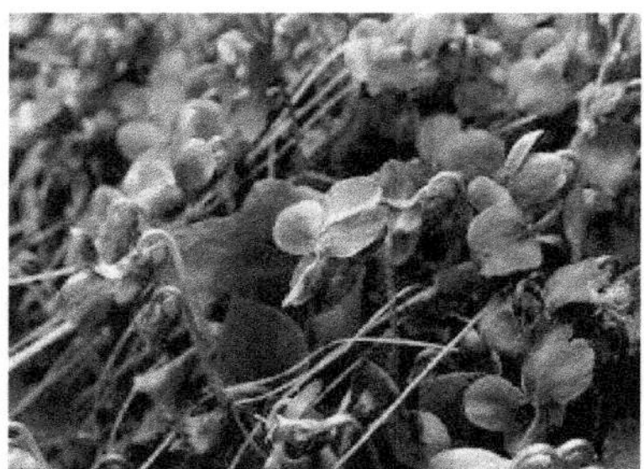

This helps with water retention, cellulite, and helps to tone the skin.

These twenty-two essential oils can be used in the preparations listed in the previous chapter as well as in other preparations as well, but first you need to understand how to mix them.

Blending Essential Oils

For every teaspoon of base oil, you can add up to six drops of essential oil. You also have to take into account how you blend the essential oils together.

If the essential oil is citrus or mint, you can use these in larger drop amounts. For example, out of 6 full drops, you can use up to three.

If the essential oil is floral or leafy, like the Rosemary and Violet Leaf, you are going to use no more than two drops when your max is six.

If the essential oil is from a root or bark, like cinnamon and carrot seed, the limit should be two drops.

This is due to their evaporation rate. Lighter oils, like your peppermint, will evaporate in a few hours and needs something to anchor it. This is where the floral, herbal, and tree oils come into play. They help give peppermint the anchor it needs to last longer in the blend.

The other problem is how to convert drops into larger measurements for larger recipes. Below is a chart that should help you with that.

1 teaspoon=100 drops of essential oil
24 teaspoons = 1 ounce

Sometimes you will run across measurements in milliliters. Here is a conversion to ounces.

118 ml = 4 ounces

It's especially important to keep in mind these measurements, because putting too much essential oils into a base blend can cause contact dermatitis. A strong tingling or burning sensation when you use a blend is a good indicator you've used too many essential oils in a recipe.

Buyer Beware

When purchasing essential oils, you have oils labeled "essential oil" and "absolute".

An absolute is still an essential oil, but the oil is extracted using a method that does not destroy the flowers from which they are made. Many flowers are too delicate to go the conventional way of getting the oils of the flower petals. This is because the petals are destroyed when intense heat is applied to them. Hence, the more delicate method is used. Because of this method, the essential oils will be more expensive.

Also, be on the lookout for essential oils that are diluted by the manufacturer. These will generally have the oil they have been diluted with on the label. There is nothing wrong with this type of marketing. They are just trying to make the essential oil or absolute more affordable. They are, however, not viable to use in recipes that call for the undiluted essential oil.

Make sure the essential you are buying comes from as close to the country of origin as possible. This is because, when the plant matter is from the country of origin, it will be more potent due to the soil being more ideal.

Also, check the average price of the essential oil on the market. This will give you a good idea of what you are going to pay.

Ask how the material used is screened for purity. The most advanced way to test is using mass spectrometer. This is a most effective way to screen for foreign chemicals in the plants that can compromise the medicinal properties.

Chapter 3 - On the Go!

The one thing you can always count on when on the road to losing weight is that the world does not stop and neither does the temptation. You need to be able to carry with you a means to stay on course. Here are a few recipes and tips you can use to help you.

Quick Tips

1.   Taking a whiff of peppermint can help you curb hunger pangs and your appetite in general. You can place three drops of this essential oil on a cotton ball and place it in a resealable bag. When the hunger hits or before you eat, take a whiff of the cotton ball.

2.   Cinnamon is also a hunger suppressant. You can use it the same way as peppermint above.

3.   You can put three drops of lemon essential oil in a glass of warm water and drink before meals to help stop cravings and increase energy levels.

4.   If you're feeling anxious or a little down on yourself, try putting three drops of either Bergamot or Grapefruit on the cotton ball above.

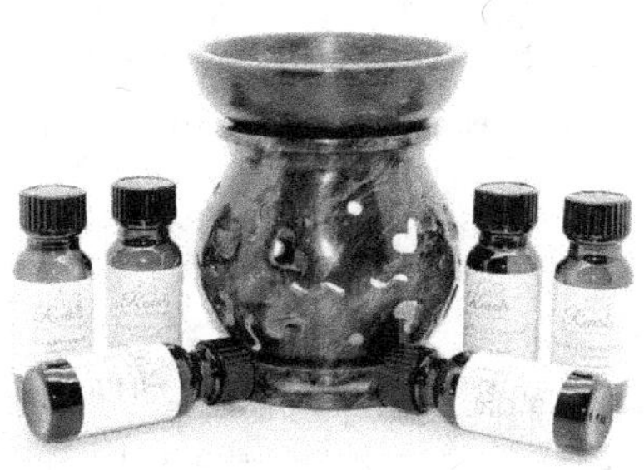

Inhaler Recipe I
(For hunger/cravings)

6 Drops of Grapefruit Essential Oil

5 Drops of Peppermint Essential Oil

4 Drops of Cinnamon Essential Oil

Inhaler Recipe II
(For fat burning)

6 Drops of Lemon Essential Oil

5 Drops of Ginger Essential Oil

4 Drops Rosemary Essential Oil

Inhaler Recipe III
(For metabolism Boosting and Water Retention)

6 Drops of Mandarin Essential Oil

5 Drops of Peppermint Essential Oil

4 Drops of Lemon Essential Oil

Diffuser Recipe I
(Cellulite/Cortisol help)

This will be more focused on alleviating stress and boosting a more calm mood. Also included will be a recipe for digestive help.

4 Drops Bergamot Essential Oil
4 Drops Violet Leaf Essential Oil
2 Drops Fennel Essential Oil

Diffuser Recipe II
(Detox and Mood Elevator)

3 Drops Grapefruit Essential Oils
3 Drops Jasmine Essential Oils
2 Drops Coriander Seed Essential Oils
2 Drops Frankincense Essential Oils

Diffuser Recipe III
(Liver and Digestion)

3 Drops of Bergamot Essential Oil
3 Drops of Coriander Seed Essential Oil
2 Drops Fennel Essential Oil
2 Drops of Greenland Moss Essential Oil

Oinment Recipe for Cellulite

25 Drops of Grapefruit Essential oil
20 Drops of Eucalyptus Peppermint Essential Oil
15 Drops of Cedarwood Essential Oil
10 Drops of Greenland Moss Essential Oil

Ointment for Metabolism and Water Retention

25 Drops of Cypress Essential Oil
20 Drops of Ginger Essential Oil
15 Drops of Carrot Seed Essential Oil
10 Cinnamon Essential Oil

Chapter 4 - Blends in the Bath

The best way to relax and kick your body into gear is to take a good old fashioned bath and just soak. This would also mean planning baths into your day. That's not a bad thing. It is one of the best ways to relieve stress.

Quick Tips

1. Always let the preparation sit for 24 hours so it can blend well.
2. You can use just one essential oil in the any of the recipes below. Just make sure it's not the wood-based or herbal ones like Rosemary, Fennel, or Coriander.

Sugar Scrub, Mineral Baths, and Bath Salt Recipes

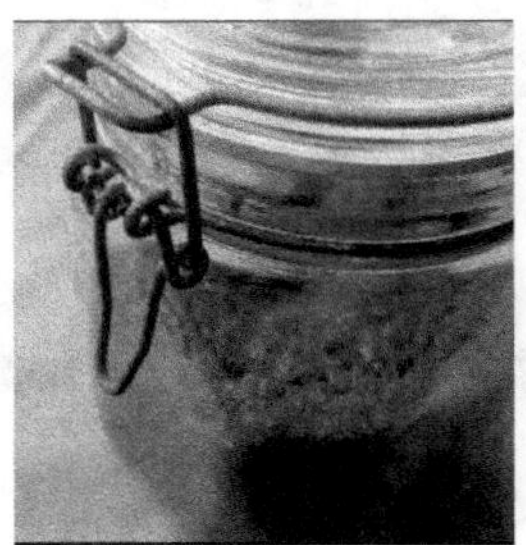

Cellulite Scrub

15 Drops of Grapefruit Essential Oil
10 Drops of Eucalyptus Essential Oil
10 Drops of Coriander Essential Oil
10 Drops of Virginia Cedarwood Essential Oil

Detox Scrub

20 Drops Lemongrass Essential Oil
15 Drops Peppermint Essential Oil
10 Drops Rosemary Essential Oil

All Purpose

You can use this one on cellulite and even swollen ankles and other places due to water retention.

15 Drops Orange Essential Oil
15 Drops Ginger Essential Oil
10 Drops Violet Leaf Essential Oil
10 Drops of Frankincense Essential Oil

Mineral Bath

It is important to note that magnesium is not as harsh as Epsom Salts and dissolves more easily in bath water. It's also good for restless leg syndrome and circulatory issues.

1 1/2 Cup Magnesium Salts
1/2 Cup Sea Salt
1/2 Cup Borax
1/4 Cup Sweet Almond Oil

Mineral Bath for Detoxing

8 Drops of Carrot Seed Essential oil
4 Drops of Coriander Essential oil
4 Drops of Cinnamon Essential oil
4 Drops of Greenland Moss Essential oil

Mineral Bath for Boosting Mood

5 Drops of Bergamot Essential Oil
5 Drops of Ginger Essential Oil
5 Drops of Orange Essential Oil
5 Drops of Frankincense Essential Oil

Bath Salts

1 1/2 Cup Epsom Salts
1/4 Cup Baking Soda
1/4 Cup Borax
1/2 Cup Sea Salt

Cellulite and Digestive

5 Drops each of:

Greenland Moss Essential Oil
Mandarin Essential Oil
Peppermint Essential Oil
Saro Essential Oil

Mood Boosting and Stress

5 Drops each of:

Bergamot Essential Oil
Frankincense Essential Oil
Grapefruit Essential Oil
Jasmine Essential Oil

Chapter 5 - Let's Get Topical

This is the chapter where we go into lotions and massage oils. Lotions and massage oils can penetrate deeper into the skin then other preparations because you have to work them into the skin.

Pre-Made Lotion Base

This is a base you can find in many places online, but I highly recommend you purchase it from brambleberry.com. I buy all my base oils and bases from there. They are very reliable and the turn-around rate from ordering to your door is great, too.

Making your own Lotion base

You may find that you are curious as to how to make lotion and not wan to buy the base at all. That is up to you. If that is your decision, here is a recipe you can cook up.

1/2 Cup of base or carrier oil
1/4 cup coconut oil
1/4 Beeswax
1 teaspoon Vitamin E oil*
2 Tablespoons Shea or Coco Butter*
(*Optional ingredients)

Instruction:

1.   In a double boiler, place all the oils and beeswax. If you have elected to use any of the butter listed above, you can add them to this step, too.

2.   Let the double boiler do its work and melt the solids.

3.   Add the Vitamin E oil after all the other ingredients have melt, if you've chosen to use it.

4.   Wait for the mixture to cool and blend in the essential oils.

5.   Place the mixture into a jar that has a tight lid. Sorry, but it won't work too well in a lotion pump bottle.

Lotions, massage oils, and Roll-ons

Cellulite Cream

(Per ounce of lotion)

15 Drops of Mandarin Essential oil
15 Drops of Grapefruit Essential Oil
10 Drops of Ginger Essential Oil
10 Drops of Virginia Cedarwood Essential Oil

Cellulite and Water Retention cream

Used in areas where swelling occurs due to water retention.
(Per 4 ounces of lotion)

15 Drops of Cypress Essential Oil
15 Drops of Virginia Cedarwood Essential Oil
10 Drops of Fennel Essential Oil
10 Drops of Carrot Seed Essential Oil

Coritsol and Stress Cream

Cortisol the is stubborn fat that hold tight to your body during times of stress.
(per 4 ounces of lotion)

15 Drops of Bergamot Essential Oil

15 Drops of Jasmine Essential Oil

10 Drops of Grapefruit Essential Oil

10 Drops of Frankincense Essential Oil

Stress Relief Massage Oil

2 Ounces Sweet Almond Oil

2 Ounces of Jojoba Oil

20 Drops of Bergamot Essential Oil

10 Drops of Jasmine Essential Oil

15 Drops of Mandarin Essential Oil

5 Drops of Carrot Seed Essential Oil

Detox Massage Oil

4 Ounces Grapeseed Oil

20 Drops of Lemongrass Essential Oil

10 Drops of Peppermint Essential Oil

10 Drops of Rosemary Essential Oil

10 Drops of Greenland Moss Essential Oil

Cellulite Massage Oil

4 Ounces of Apricot Oil

20 Drops of Grapefruit Essential Oil

10 Drops of Lemon Essential Oil

10 Drops of Ginger Essential Oil

10 Drops of Coriander Seed Essential Oil

Roll-ons

These are on-the-go versions of massage oils. They are small, compact, and can be applied any time of the day for periodic application or to help avoid those cravings.

Citrus Shot for Appetite/Cravings

Apply under the nose.

2 Ounces Grapeseed oil
10 Drops Grapefruit Essential Oil
10 Drops Orange Essential Oil
5 Drops Lemon Essential Oil

Tummy Tonic

Apply to wrists and take a deep breath. You can also apply to the abdominal section.

2 Ounces Sweet Almond Oil
10 Drops Peppermint Essential Oil
10 Drops Bergamot Essential Oil
5 Drops Fennel Essential Oil

Stress Shot

Apply to temples and base of the skull in the back of the head.

10 Drops Jasmine Essential Oil
10 Drops Mandarin Essential Oil
5 Drops Frankincense Essential Oil

Chapter 6 - Can I Cook with These?

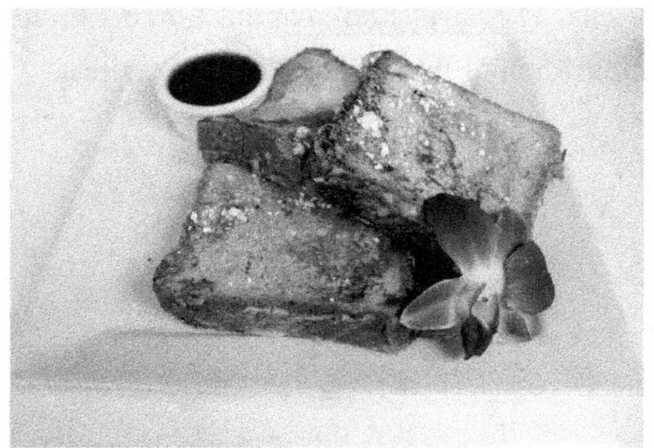

Here is probably the hardest topic in the realm of essential oils, but yes, you can cook with them. You just don't use as much of the essential oil as you would the actual herb you would normally cook with. From breakfast to desserts, yes, desserts, you can add essential oils to just about anything. Here are a few substitutions and a little treat to cap it off.

French Toast Dredge

2 Eggs
4 Drops Cinnamon Essential Oil
2 Drops Orange Essential Oil
1/4 tsp Vanilla Extract

Hot Cocoa

1 tablespoon Hershey's Cocoa
6 Ounces Coconut Milk
1/4 tsp Vanilla Extract
6 Drops of Peppermint

Rosemary Vinaigrette

1 tsp Balsamic Vinegar

3 tsp Olive Oil

4 Drops Rosemary Essential Oil

4 Drops Orange Essential Oil

Just a little Lemon

1 tsp Balsamic Vinegar

1 tsp Olive Oil

2 tsp Grapeseed Oil

8 Drops Lemon Essential Oil

Strawberry Peppermint Water

8 Ounces of Filtered Water

1/2 Cup of chopped strawberries

4 Drops of Peppermint Essential Oil

1. Place the strawberries in a small pitcher

2. Pour the water into the pitcher

3. Add the essential oil.

4. Using a wooden spoon, mash the strawberries to get the juice out.

5. Add 1 tsp honey if you like

Let it chill for a couple of hours before shaking well and drinking.

Orange Coconut Ice Cream

(2) 13.5 Ounce cans of coconut milk with the fat

1 1/2 tablespoons of Arrowroot powder

Pinch of Sea salt

1/2 Cup Raw Honey or Organic Maple Syrup

1/4 teaspoon Vanilla Extract

4 Drops of Orange or Mandarin Essential Oil

Instruction:

1.   Mix the two cans of coconut milk together until blended.

2.   Reserve a 1/4 cup of the milk and heat the rest.

3.   Add the Arrowroot powder to the 1/4 cup of milk. Whisk until dissolved.

4.   Whisk the warm milk into the Arrowroot mixture until it thickens.

5.   Whisk in remaining ingredients.

6.   Let chill for a couple of hours before making it the rest of the way in an ice cream maker.

Conclusion

I hope this book has helped you a lot in getting your feet wet with essential oils and their uses. May you have the best luck with your new, healthy life style. Until Next time.